POUND SALT:

101 Simple Tips for Eating Low Sodium, Finding the Sodium in Food, Reducing Your Salt Intake, Giving Up High Sodium Foods, and Lowering the Chance of Disease Caused By a High Sodium Diet

BY: CLW GUIDES

CONTENTS

INTRODUCTION

Americans are consuming more and more salt in their diets, resulting in high blood pressure, heart disease, and many other conditions. If you've been told to limit your salt intake, it may be confusing where to begin since practically everything that tastes good contains salt. This handy guide will give you a brief background on sodium: what foods contain it and how it can affect you. Then, you will discover 101 fast and easy tips to help you start reducing your sodium intake right away!

What is Sodium?

Sodium is an essential nutrient most commonly found in sodium chloride or table salt. It occurs naturally in many foods, including milk, fruits, and vegetables, but it is also added to processed and packaged foods in higher amounts as a preservative and a flavor enhancer. Processed foods can contain several forms of sodium, including sodium nitrite, baking soda, sodium benzoate, sodium saccharine, and monosodium glutamate, or MSG. Broth, condiments, sauces, processed meats, and canned foods almost always contain added sodium, many in dangerously high amounts.

On average, about 75 percent of the sodium we eat comes from processed, packaged, and restaurant foods. About 12 percent comes from foods with natural sodium like vegetables, and about 10 percent comes from table salt that we add to food during or after cooking.

Why is Sodium Essential to your Body?

A moderate amount of sodium is needed to stay in good health. The body uses sodium for many important functions, including regulating blood pressure. Sodium dissolves in the blood and holds water, which maintains the essential liquid in the blood. It also helps sustain the body's hydration levels, especially for people who exercise frequently or who work outside in the heat.

Sodium helps transmit electrical signals throughout the body, which is essential for muscle and nerve functioning. Before muscles contract, sodium triggers an electrical signal that causes the muscle fibers to shorten. Without sodium, the muscles would have difficulty working, and the nervous system would work less efficiently.

Salt and sodium also play a role in the production of stomach acid, which lets the body absorb nutrients and kill bacteria.

What Happens if you Don't Get Enough Sodium?

The body doesn't need much sodium to function, so it's very rare to have a sodium deficiency. However, low sodium, or hyponatremia, can occur. Hyponatremia is usually caused by an imbalance of water and sodium levels in the blood, either because of an excess of water or because of a lack of sodium.

Extreme athletes are at a greater risk of developing hyponatremia because intense exercise can rid the body of sodium. The condition also can occur as a result of medical conditions or symptoms, including vomiting, kidney disease, liver disease, hypothyroidism, and some medications. Hyponatremia can also affect older people and those living in a hot climate.

The most common symptoms of hyponatremia include weakness, fatigue, nausea, headache, muscle cramps, and irritability. More severe symptoms include confusion, hallucinations, and coma. The treatment for the condition varies depending on the cause, but it usually focuses on restoring the balance of water and sodium in the blood. Individuals with the condition may need to adjust their medications or use an IV sodium solution.

What Happens if you Get Too Much Sodium?

Consuming more sodium than your body needs is much more common than not getting enough salt. Sodium intake tends to correlate with blood pressure, so if you consume too much sodium, it can lead to hypertension. Sodium in the blood holds water, so when there's an excess of sodium, your body develops too much water in your blood, which causes the volume of your blood to increase. Because blood vessels can't expand, your blood pressure rises.

High blood pressure increases your risk for many other conditions, including heart disease, heart failure, stroke, and kidney damage. It's responsible for two-thirds of all strokes and half of all heart disease cases.

Consuming too much sodium can also increase your risk of stomach cancer, according to the World Cancer Research Fund. Salt can damage your stomach lining, which can cause lesions. When left untreated, these lesions could eventually turn into stomach cancer.

Excessive sodium may lead to osteoporosis as well.

Several studies have found a potential link between salt intake and calcium levels in your blood. A high salt intake can cause your body to lose calcium through urination. Then, your body will replace this lost calcium with calcium from the bones, which can lead to osteoporosis.

Finally, when your body takes in too much salt, it will retain water to counteract the effects. This will very often cause you to gain weight. Extra pounds contribute to the likelihood of developing all of the health conditions described in this section. To make matters worse, excess salt in your diet will very likely make it even more difficult to lose weight when you finally commit to it.

What is the Recommended Sodium Intake?

The average adult should consume a maximum of 2,300 milligrams of sodium per day, which is equivalent to the amount of sodium in one teaspoon of salt, or a single box of convenience macaroni and cheese. Some people should only consume up to 1,500 milligrams per day, including older adults and those with high blood sugar. The Office of Disease Prevention and Health also suggests that African Americans consume less than 1,500 milligrams per day because they are at a greater risk of developing high blood pressure at a younger age.

Because of the prevalence of packaged and processed foods, almost all Americans consume too much salt for decades without realizing it, until health problems present themselves. Most of this excess sodium comes from processed foods, but some comes from using a salt shaker during meals. On average, Americans consume 3,500 milligrams of sodium per day, which is almost 150 percent of the recommended daily intake.

Some foods contain a high percentage of the recommended daily sodium intake in just one serving. For example, one cup of spaghetti sauce has about 1,200 milligrams of sodium, one can of chicken noodle soup has about 1,100 milligrams, and one tablespoon of teriyaki sauce has almost 700 milligrams.

How Can you Lower Sodium Intake?

Many people know that it is time to tell sodium to Pound Salt and finally commit to a lower salt diet. However, because sodium is added to so many foods before you buy them, it can be a challenging goal. Consuming a balanced amount of sodium is essential for your health, and it is possible to accomplish with some effort.

This guide is a great place to begin. Turn the page for 101 tips for reducing your sodium intake right now!

101 TIPS TO REDUCE YOUR SODIUM

1 – KNOW YOUR NUMBERS

1.   A person needs approximately 500 mg of sodium a day to survive unless they are extremely active during the day.

2.   The average American consumes 3,500 mg or more a day.

3.   The American Heart Association recommends a maximum daily intake of 1,500 -2,000 mg of sodium.

4.   A heart healthy food should have no more than 480 mg of sodium per serving. Meal products should have no more than 600 mg of sodium per serving. Even those sodium counts will add up quickly when trying to fit your diet into the recommended daily intake of 1,500-2,000 mg. Try to avoid processed foods as much as possible as the sodium content of fresh foods is substantially lower than for processed foods.

2 – KNOW THE MYTHS VS THE FACTS

5.   **Myth**: You should eliminate sodium completely for optimum health.

Fact: All of the adverse effects of sodium in your diet might suggest that you should remove salt completely. However, sodium is an essential nutrient that controls your blood pressure and helps nerves and muscles to work properly. It contributes to the processing of regular water intake as well. The problem is, however, that most people choose foods containing substantially more sodium than they need. Your body only needs about 500 mg of salt per day to be healthy. Many reach that amount of salt before their breakfast is complete.

6.   **Myth:** On a hot day or during routine exercise where you sweat, you need more salt in your diet.

Fact: The percentage of salt lost through sweat is minor, so there is no need to consume extra salt, although it is important to drink a lot of liquids, especially water.

7.   **Myth:** You only need to worry about your salt levels if you have high blood pressure.

Fact: Lowering your intake of salt now will reduce the chances of developing high blood pressure or other health conditions such as kidney disease in the future.

8.   **Myth:** Only old people need to worry about salt intake.

Fact: Research study after research study supports the findings that excess sodium can negatively affect children and teens as well as adults. At the 2017 Pediatric Academic Societies Meeting in May, 2017, a study funded by the National Institutes of Health was presented that gave strong evidence that excess salt in a teens diet leads to premature hardening of the arteries, a symptom of heart disease. The incidents of high blood pressure in teens and children have substantially increased in recent years, as has the amount of sodium in the average child's diet. High sodium effects bone, brain, stomach, and kidney health as well.

While it's true that some people who are at a greater risk of developing high blood pressure need to be more careful about sodium intake than others, too much sodium can be a problem for anyone. It's a misconception that only older people or people with high blood sugar need to watch their sodium intake. In reality, people of all ages should be careful with sodium, regardless of their medical history or health conditions. Everyone can improve their health and reduce their risk of high blood pressure and heart disease by keeping their sodium intake within the healthy range.

9.   **Myth:** Sodium is only found in foods.

Fact: Some over the counter and prescription medications contain sodium as well. Read drug labels as carefully as you read food labels.

10: **Myth:** I don't cook with salt or salt my food so I don't have a problem with high sodium.

Fact: More than 75% of the sodium people consume comes not from adding salt while cooking or at the table, but from processed and restaurant food.

11. **Myth:** Sea Salt and Kosher salt have less

sodium than table salt.

Fact: Salt is salt. Regardless of where the salt comes from, the sodium in the salt is responsible for adverse health effects.

12. **Myth:** Foods high in salt taste salty.

Fact: Some foods that are high in sodium don't taste salty because they are mixed with other spices or ingredients that mask the taste. Also, your brain and body have been conditions over many years to register foods high in salt as normal. You can't really know how much salt you are consuming without reading food labels to find out sodium levels.

13. **Myth:** Food tastes too bland if there is no added salt to enhance the flavor.

Fact: Food does not need salt to be satisfying. There are many low-sodium alternatives to spice up the flavor of your food. And, gradually lowering the content of salt in your diet can decrease your desire for salty food over time. It may take some time to adjust, but you may find you enjoy a wider range of foods and flavors than you did when you relied on salt to spice up your food.

3 – CUT BACK GRADUALLY

14. **It Takes Time** – Give yourself time to get used to food with lower salt. As with any new habit, expect it to take from 6 to 8 weeks. Small steps will get you there eventually, and you will find that as you make lower-sodium choices more and more often, that you will crave lower salt foods.

15. **Cut Back Gradually** – Decrease your use of salt gradually. As you transition, combine a lower salt version with a conventional product. For example, rather than going cold turkey with salt-free peanut butter, use half salt-free and half regular peanut butter until you get used to the lower salt taste. Gradually decrease the amount of the conventional product until you enjoy the low or no salt version on its own. This method works especially well with condiments (ketchup, mustard, etc.), jarred pasta sauces and

broths.

16. **Use Less** – If you must include salt in a recipe, add the next smallest measurement than called for in the recipe. For example, if a recipe asks for 1 tsp of salt, add ½ tsp instead. Sometimes, you can omit added salt in a recipe altogether. Reducing the amount you add will rarely diminish your enjoyment of the dish.

17. **Eat Smaller Portion Sizes** – Smaller amounts result in less salt, even if you are eating a high sodium food. Choose lots of fresh fruits and veggies, which contain virtually no salt, to supplement a smaller portion of a larger sodium dish.

18. **Substitute** – You may want to consider a salt substitute, which, unless you have a medical reason to limit your potassium, you can shake more freely than salt. Salt substitutes replace some or all of the salt with potassium. Check with your doctor before using a salt substitute to make sure the potassium won't counteract with medication or harm a particular medical condition. Many people enjoy salt substitutes and notice no apparent difference from the real thing, while others are less enamored and think the taste is off. At any rate, if you are a salt-a-holic, a salt substitute may help to reduce your consumption.

19. **Add At-Home Meals** – Slowly wean

yourself from eating in restaurants or eating prepackaged meals and spend more time planning and preparing your meals. As one takeout fast food meal can contain up to 1,500 mg OR MORE of sodium, merely reducing the number of times you rely on "fast food" can help control your salt intake.

20. **Fresh First** – Choose a fresh ingredient (e.g., corn off the cob) over a processed one (canned corn), which can shave tons of sodium off your meal. You will eventually even find yourself enjoying the taste of meals made with fresh ingredients more than those previously prepared with packaged contents.

21. **Write it Down** – If you want to reduce your sodium but don't know where you are taking in the most, journal everything you eat for one week and then calculate how much sodium you are consuming. Use your journal to discover where you are eating too much sodium and look for smart swaps to replace those trigger foods (see the SMART SWAPS section below for ideas).

22. **Get Help** – You may want to consider engaging a dietician to help you to analyze your diet and make a plan to reduce your sodium intake.

4 – IN THE GROCERY STORE

23. **Read Product Labels on all Processed Foods –** Look for products with 300 mg of sodium or less per individual serving.

24. **Know What Product Labels Mean Relating to Salt –**

Sodium free: less than 5 mg per serving

Very low Sodium: less than 35 mg per serving

Low sodium: 140 mg or less

Reduced sodium: 25 percent less sodium than usual

Light in sodium: 50 percent less sodium than usual

Unsalted; without salt added; or no salt added: contains only the salt that naturally appears in food

25. **The Many Names of Salt** – Be aware that food labels use different names for sodium, but all mean salt in your food! Here are some common names and descriptions you may encounter for sodium:

Monosodium glutamate (MSG)

Baking powder

Baking soda

Brine

Disodium 5

Disodium EDTA

Disodium phosphate

Guanylate

Salt

Sodium alginate

Sodium bicarbonate

Sodium benzoate

Sodium chloride

Sodium citrate

Sodium erythorbate

Sodium metabisulfite

Sodium nitrite

Sodium propionate

Sodium saccharin

26. **They Are Not All the Same** – Compare several brands of the same food item until you find the one with the lowest sodium content. Sodium levels vary widely between the same or similar grocery products. Keep in mind the number of servings noted on the container when deciding the best option.

27. **Choose Wisely** – When available, choose canned goods and other staples labeled as low, reduced, or no salt versions.

28. **Know What to Avoid** – Stay clear of canned, cured, salted or smoked meat. All these types of meat use substantial amounts of salt in their processing.

29. **Hidden Salt in Meat Products** – Many types of meat and poultry have injections of salt solutions as a preservative. Make sure to look at the packaging and ingredient list to see if there are added preservatives. The packaging may reference that the meat packed in broth, saline or sodium solution or one of the descriptions for sodium noted in #25 above will appear on the ingredient list. Consider a

different brand if you see sodium added in this way.

30. **Fresh Tastes Best** – Choose the freshest fruits and vegetables you can find. Fresh produce tastes better and doesn't need salt added for great flavor.

31. **AHA Seal** – Look for products with the American Heart Association's heart smart check mark. The check mark tells a shopper that the product has passed the American Heart Association's test as a healthy heart choice. While their stamp of approval doesn't guarantee that the product is low in salt, it is a good product choice to start with when doing your label checks.

5 – IN THE KITCHEN

32. **Add Salt at the Right Time –** Never add salt to boiling water when cooking pasta, veggies, rice, cereal or potatoes. Wait to add it to a dish when the impact is strongest—at the end of cooking or, better yet, at the table. When sprinkled on just before serving, the flavoring goes farther.

33. **Avoid Stacking Salty Foods –** For instance, if a recipe calls for cheese, you likely do not need to add salt as well, because cheese already contains salt. If your dish contains an ingredient already high in sodium, lighten up on other salty seasonings or ingredients.

34. **Look for Great Tasting Substitutes –** For instance, try fresh cucumbers rather than pickles. If you absolutely must include that high salt

ingredient, make sure to balance your recipe with lower salt options.

35. **Always Measure** – When cooking with sodium laden seasonings and other ingredients, always measure. You cannot rely on your eyes to determine a proper measurement. If a recipe calls for salt or another high sodium item, consider reducing the salt content by cutting down the amount of that particular ingredient. You will likely not notice a difference and that small activity alone can substantially reduce the sodium content in your dish.

36. **Try to Cook from Scratch** – And use the freshest ingredients possible. Processed foods are usually drenched in salt and can blow your sodium budget fast.

37. **Use Frozen Veggies** – Frozen vegetables are typically lower in salt than canned. Make sure to choose frozen vegetables that are not sauced or seasoned and double check the sodium content on the label to be safe.

38. **Drain and Rinse** – If you must use canned goods, draining and rinsing them can reduce the sodium content by up to 40%. Rinsing is an especially helpful trick if using canned beans, as cooking beans from scratch is a significant time investment.

39. **Water it Down** – Dilute reduced sodium

broth with water or wine to reduce the salt content.

40. **Limit Convenience Mixes** – Hamburger Helper, flavored rice packets or boxes and noodle packages are all high in sodium. Consider preparing extra rice when cooking a meal and freezing the leftovers for a quick, low-salt addition to a future meal.

41. **Try Adding Acid** – Adding acidic flavorings when cooking instead of salt enhances the flavor of food without added sodium. Lemon juice, lime juice, and vinegar all are salt-free. A sprinkle of lemon, lime, or orange zest can boost the flavor of a dish as well, without having to add unwanted sodium.

42. **Call on Herbs** – Chopped fresh herbs, garlic, shallots, and onions can enhance a dish's flavor without adding salt.

43. **Salt-Free Seasonings** – Many dried herbs and seasoning blends are salt-free and can be used to replace unhealthy sodium in your cooking. Be careful to check labels before buying, but these salt-free seasonings are a straightforward and convenient way to cut back on salt.

44. **Roast Vegetables** – Many people find the flavor of vegetables to be harsh without added salt. Try roasting or grilling your vegetables to counteract the bitter flavors. These cooking methods enhance

the vegetable's natural sweetness and provide an appealing and tasty side dish.

45. **Cooking Method Matter** – Grilling, braising, roasting, sautéing and searing are the best cooking methods to enhance natural flavor without added salt.

46. **L-Glutamate** – Use foods that are high in L-Glutamate which triggers our taste receptors and make food taste great without added salt. These foods include mushrooms, seaweed, tomatoes, cabbage, and carrots.

47. **Fatten Up** – Healthy fats can help to enhance flavor without having to add salt. Consider roasted nuts and avocados, olive, canola, soybean or sesame seed oils.

48. **Go International** – Try cooking methods from the global community – Asian, African, Mediterranean and European. Incorporating unusual food combinations and cooking strategies give every meal exciting flavors without having to resort to boring table salt.

49. **Find Flavor From the Sea** – Using seaweed (such as kelp) instead of salt when cooking enhances the foods flavor without high sodium.

6 – AT THE TABLE

50. **Avoid Table Salt** – Don't keep a salt shaker on your dinner table, or you'll be tempted to shake salt on everything. Be mindful of using as little salt as possible when seasoning a bland dish. Sprinkle lightly, taste, and only sprinkle more if necessary. We often add so much salt to our plates that we don't realize how much sodium we're adding to our diet.

51. **Go Cold Turkey** – Although it was suggested earlier to ease into salt reduction gradually, eliminating excess salt altogether is possible, and sometimes essential, for many people. At first, your food might taste a bit bland in comparison. But once you grow used to your new diet, you'll realize that you will not crave as much salt as you did before. In fact, salty foods might eventually seem almost inedible to you.

52. Check the Lid on Your Saltshaker – This might sound like common sense, but it's all too easy for the lid to pop off and spill salt all over your plate. Since no one likes to waste food, you may find yourself eating it anyway. Make sure the lid is screwed on tightly to prevent accidents that can lead to unordinary high intakes of salt.

53. Taste Your Food Before Adding Salt – Many of us are so used to adding salt to our dishes that we sprinkle it on before we even take a bite. If you don't add salt, you might be pleasantly surprised to find that many dishes don't need it. In fact, the salt might even be overpowering the natural flavors of the dish. If your dish does require salt, add only as much as necessary, and not a single bit more.

54. Experiment with Different Spices – Instead of reaching for the salt shaker, try different herbs and spices like dry mustard, dill, nutmeg, rosemary, onion powder, etc. Don't forget about the pepper shaker! By trying different spices, you can add more variety to your diet and reduce your sodium intake. You might even find that some spices taste better than salt--and they're healthier, too.

55. Try Eating Smaller Portions – If you're trying to reduce your fat or caloric intake, you might already be doing this. So much food is loaded with sodium, especially canned and processed foods. When you eat smaller portions, you'll be taking in less salt.

56. Put Fresh Foods Onto Your Plate – Most of us load up our plates with canned vegetables – corn, peas, mashed potatoes, carrots. What many people don't realize is that canned foods are loaded with sodium. To reduce your sodium intake, try replacing canned fruits and vegetables with fresh ones. They might have a shorter shelf life, but they're just as delicious and offer more health benefits.

57. Avoid Using a Lot of Condiments – Many of us don't realize it, but condiments like ketchup and mayonnaise contain a lot of sodium. Instead of drizzling lots of sauces over your burger and fries, try limiting the amount to a teaspoon or two. Additionally, choose condiments that are lower in sodium like mustard and horseradish.

58. Keep the Salad Dressing to a Minimum – Condiments, dressings and sauces can be loaded with sodium. Even a small amount can ruin your diet if you're not careful. If you're eating a dish that requires it, serve it on the side and dip your fork in it instead of pouring. A little dressing can go a long way.

59. Include Foods Rich in Potassium – Potassium counteracts the effect of sodium. These foods include sweet potatoes, salad greens, tomatoes, white or kidney beans, oranges, bananas, and cantaloupe.

60. **Cut Back on Bread** — It is hard to believe because it doesn't usually taste salty, but bread and grain contribute an enormous amount of sodium to our diet. Yes, unfortunately, bagels, croissants, doughnuts, rolls, pastries, and hamburger and hot dog buns are all part of the bread and grain category as well. Salt is needed to help bread rise, so even multigrain and wheat bread can be full of salt. Make sure to check the labels before digging into the bread basket, and consider replacing that roll with a tasty fruit or vegetable instead.

7 – EATING OUT

61. Research the Restaurant Beforehand – Before you make plans on going to any restaurant or food establishment, research the types of foods that they serve there. If you intend on going to a restaurant that serves burgers, you will know that many of the condiments served there are high in sodium. If you plan on going to a restaurant that serves Asian cuisine, you will be aware that many of the dishes contain soy sauce, which is high in sodium. It's best to plan ahead than to be surprised.

62. Bring Your Condiments or Get them on the Side – If you intend on going to a place that has condiments with high sodium levels, bring in some low-sodium choices from home. If you can't do this, ask the restaurant to give you the condiments on the side so that you can use them sparingly. Even better, try to avoid condiments altogether if possible.

63. Order Dishes With Vegetables – If there are few low sodium meals at the restaurant, order a salad or pack your meal with plenty of vegetables, which will help to give your dish flavor without having to add unnecessary sodium to it. Be wary of salads, however, as they usually contain dressings that can be high in sodium.

64. Add Different Spices and Flavors – Although salt does add flavor to bland dishes, ask the waiter for a different spice such as pepper or paprika. You can even use fruits such as lemons or limes. There are plenty of sodium-free ways to make your dish more flavorful.

65. Know Which Foods Are High in Sodium – You should just avoid certain restaurants if you are trying to cut down on sodium. Be knowledgeable about which types of foods have high sodium levels, such as ham and pickles, and base your restaurant choice around that information.

66. Consider Going to a Small Restaurant – It is harder to request specially prepared foods from chain restaurants. Instead of going to a large chain restaurant, consider instead eating out at a small, family owned, restaurant where they will be able to prepare your food the way that you want it.

67. **Don't Be Afraid to Ask** – When it comes to food, don't be afraid to ask how food is prepared or to have your food prepared a certain way. The waiters should be able to tell you about the food and should be able to cater to your needs on most occasions. Always request "no MSG" when ordering at any sit down restaurant. Asking is necessary if you want to avoid sodium.

68. **If You Ask for Dessert, Keep it Simple** – If you decide that you want dessert, keep it limited to something made from fruit, which will prevent you from eating too much sodium. However, still ask about how their desserts are made to avoid unexpected salt in your dessert.

69. **Eat Out With Someone Who Is Also Sodium-Conscious** – If you choose to dine with someone who is also conscious of their sodium intake, you will have a better chance of avoiding and resisting foods that are high in sodium. After all, support is a great motivator to follow through.

70. **Plain Jane** – Some restaurants, such as hamburger places, have very few low-sodium options on their menu. In that case, make your dish as plain as possible. Get a hamburger without any toppings or condiments, which will lessen your sodium intake while still giving you something to eat.

71. **Select a Restaurant with Nutrition Information** – Some places are already transparent about the nutrition value of their food. If there is a place near you that has this type of information readily available, go there to make food selection easier for you.

72. **Keep Sodium Levels Low Throughout the Day** – If you know that you are going to go out to eat, track your sodium intake throughout the day and keep it as low as possible. When you go out to eat later, you can consume a higher amount of sodium, knowing you have had less than normal throughout the day.

8 – SMART SWAPS

73. Swap Potato Chips with Dried Fruit Chips – Potato chips are famously high in salt, and just about everyone is guilty of eating them at one time or another. Dried fruit chips like apple or banana chips can be just as snackable as regular potato chips but without all that extra salt.

74. Swap Pretzels with Rice Cakes – Pretzels are covered in salt, and they have a knack for inducing thirst just like the saltiest of snacks. Rice cakes have almost no sodium, and they make a great substitute for pretzels.

75. Swap Salted Peanuts with Other Nuts – Of course, something with the word 'salted' in the name is going to be high in salt, but nuts are not equal. Pistachios have little or no salt. They're a bit pricier and harder to eat, but they're also delicious and nutritious. Walnuts and Almonds are easy to find with no salt added as well.

76. **Swap Canned Soups with Homemade Soups** — Most canned food products have high salt since salt is such an effective preservative, and canned soups are a primary culprit. Try making homemade soup instead for a much healthier and better-tasting option.

77. **Swap Soy Sauce with Herbs and Spices** — Soy Sauce is all salt, which is why it's so delicious, but your favorite herbs and spices can be just as yummy when applied correctly. Garlic is a great place to start.

78. **Swap Deli Ham with Sliced Chicken** — Almost all deli meats have high levels of sodium, but chicken and roast beef tend to have less. Freshly cooked, non-preserved chicken sliced thin is one of the best options for sandwich meat.

79. **Swap Cheese with Lettuce** — Despite the brilliant deliciousness of cheese, it is often unnecessary in many foods. When making a sandwich, try swapping the slice of cheese with a leaf of lettuce.

80. **Swap Cheddar or American Cheese**

with Swiss Cheese – Swiss cheese contains only 50-60 mg of salt per serving compared to up to 200 mg for other cheese types.

81. **Swap Salad Dressing with Oil and Vinegar –** Very few store-bought salad dressings are low in sodium, but mixing oil and vinegar allows you to remove the salt content completely. If you already favor oil-based dressings, the swap is easy!

82. **Swap Ketchup with Homemade Salsa –** Ketchup is loaded with both salt and sugar, and, surprisingly, little tomato. Homemade salsa is quick to make and much healthier. It can also be much tastier, and making it from scratch lets you season it to taste.

83. **Swap Mayonnaise with Hummus –** Hummus makes a great alternative for those who hate dry sandwiches. You can even use it as a substitute for mayo in baked recipes or casseroles.

84. **Swap Peanut Butter with Salt-Free Peanut Butter –** This one is fairly obvious, but regular peanut butter has a ton of sodium as a preservative. Salt-free peanut butter is smooth, creamy, and much tastier than what most people believe. It doesn't have as long a shelf life, but it doesn't stay on the shelf long anyway!

85. **Swap Mustard with Vinegar –** For some,

it's hard to imagine a sandwich without that bitter tang of mustard. Unfortunately, even though it contains less sodium than ketchup or mayonnaise, it has way too much salt for a condiment. Vinegar is a great substitute, and there are multiple varieties to choose from, including apple, wine, and rice.

86. **Swap Bottled Spaghetti Sauce with Homemade Spaghetti Sauce** – Most sauces of any sort that come in a bottle or can have far too much sodium. Homemade spaghetti sauce is relatively easy to make, and it doesn't take much time. Fresh ingredients are always better than preserved, but if you need to use canned, look for salt-free versions of tomatoes and tomato sauce, and substitute other spices for the bottled salt.

87. **Swap French Fries with Baked Veggies** – The potato portion of the French fry itself isn't very high in sodium, but most French fries come doused in salt, especially the frozen varieties. Try baking carrot sticks or Zucchini with some pepper and garlic instead.

88. **Swap Pizza with Fresh Pasta** – Pizza is all high-sodium ingredients, but if you want the Italian experience, pasta is the way to go. Don't add salt when cooking the pasta, and use your homemade spaghetti sauce to create a perfect Italian-inspired meal.

89. **Swap Popcorn with Unsalted Popcorn**

— Thanks to movie theaters and ballparks, people expect their popcorn to be incredibly salty, and most store-bought brands reflect that in their ingredients. Choose an unsalted option instead for the classic snack experience without the danger. Or, experiment with salt free seasonings on your popcorn instead.

90. **Swap Canned Beans with Fresh Beans**

— Canned foods, in general, have so much sodium that they shouldn't be an option unless there is no other choice. Always search for fresh, non-frozen versions in the produce section, including raw beans. Dried beans are excellent as well.

91. **Swap Pickles with Cucumbers** — Pickles

are the one type of pickled food that doesn't say the name of what is pickled, but pickles are just pickled cucumbers. Raw cucumbers are crisp and light, and they are perfect with a light vinegar coat when sliced for sandwiches.

92. **Swap Salt with Pepper** — Salt and Pepper

are a pair that goes together so well almost every table in America has them both side by side. They are just as good used individually. If you're trying to cut back on the salt, give your food a little kick of pepper instead.

93. **Swap Frozen Dinners with Fresh**

Meals – Frozen foods of just about all varieties have high sodium levels, so try to prepare homemade versions of the same meals you enjoy frozen. You'll find the fresh versions taste much better, and they are better for you.

94. Swap Processed Meats with Farm-Fresh

– Just because processed meats are high in sodium doesn't mean all meats are. There are tons of farm-fresh meats that never receive any preservatives, even salt. Look for these in the butcher section of your grocery store.

95. Swap Buttermilk with Yogurt

– Buttermilk has a surprising amount of salt, but yogurt lacks that extra ingredient. Most recipes that call for buttermilk will easily allow for the substitution of plain yogurt.

96. Swap Cottage Cheese with Cream Cheese

– Certain dairy products, like cottage cheese, have a lot of salt, but others, like cream cheese, do not. Cream cheese is a relatively standard substitute for cottage cheese.

97. Swap Croutons with Baked Breadsticks

– Packaged croutons are not too different from potato chips, but you can make a version at home with very little salt at all. Cut low salt breadsticks and bake them until they turn brown, then cut them into small squares.

98. Swap Instant Pudding with Stove-Top Pudding

– Instant pudding has a ridiculous amount of sodium, and the stove-top pudding option lacks that salt. It takes a bit more effort, but it's well worth it.

99. Swap Salted Butter with Vegetable Oil

– Vegetable oil is an excellent substitute for salted butter or margarine, and it works about the same in most dishes.

100. Swap Canned Olives for Fresh Olives –

Canned olives are similar to pickled veggies as they have massive amounts of salt as a preservative. Fresh olives are just as tasty but without all that added salt.

101. Swap Salted Bread Rolls for Fresh Bread

– Most prepackaged bread rolls are either made with tons of salt or covered in a light coating of it after coming out of the oven. Seek out unsalted fresh bread from your grocery store's bakery.

CONCLUSION

It can be hard to say Pound Salt to sodium and switch to lower-salt foods, but the health benefits are worth it. And, after a while, your desire for salt will decrease. Most people who lower their sodium intake find that it takes two or more months to adjust. Eventually, however, you won't miss sodium at all. In fact, foods with lots of salt, like potato chips, will taste overwhelmingly salty after you adjust to a lower-sodium diet.

Gradually work through the 101 tips listed in this guide, and soon you will find reducing your salt content is no problem at all!

Dear Reader:

We hope you enjoyed this book and found a lot of helpful tips and tricks for reducing sodium in your diet. Choose the ones you want to apply and skip those you don't like, to suit your personal nutrition strategy.

We work hard to provide quality guides, so if you've spotted a typo please email us at CLWGuides@gmail.com.

Amazon Reviews are very welcome. Email us the link to your review and **we will send you a free review copy of another CLW guide**. Getting reviews for our guides is a big deal and we look forward to hearing what you think. If possible, mention which tip you found most helpful and why.

CLW Guides – Compressed Learning Worth Something

Our goal is to save you hours of internet research by providing high quality concise guides on topics of interest to you.